Become a Nurse
&
Work in United States

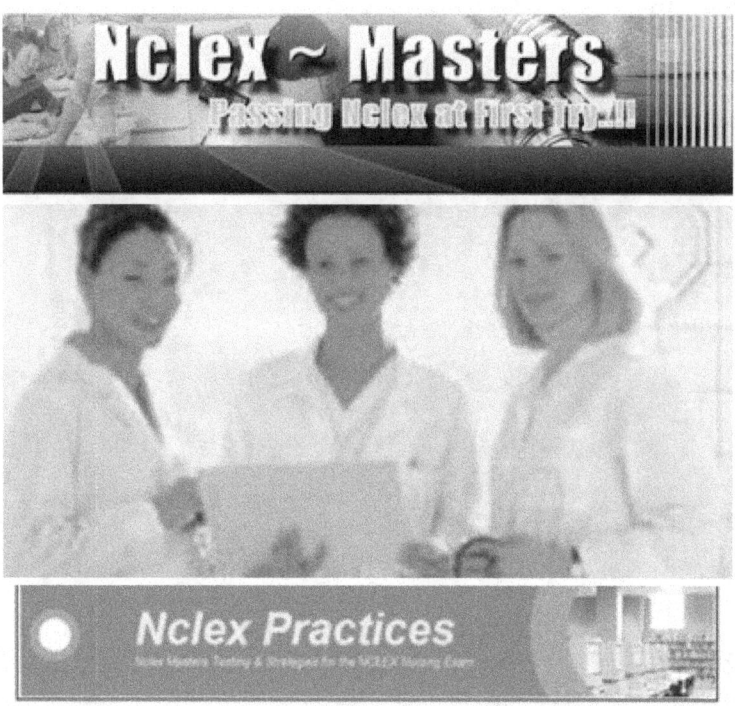

FREE Online Exam Prep 99% NCLEX Format

Ten Steps Guide
for
International Nurses

First Edition by NCLEX Masters

Copyrighted USA 2008

Becoming a Registered Nurse in United States is a long and complex process.
 Know All Steps and Sub-Steps to succeed. Each of the steps below may have other sub-steps and information all internationally educated nurses need to successfully become a Registered Nurse in United States.

1. **Credentialing**
   a. Search education credentialing services & save
   b. Submit credentialing request
   c. Contact your nursing school ~ Mail the documentation yourself
   d. Follow up online with access ID
2. **RN Application**
   a. Contact nursing boards – State selection
   b. Request or download application forms
   c. Wait for ATT and Pearson-Vue
3. **NCLEX registration**
   a. Pearson-Vue and NCLEX
   b. Register for NCLEX exam
   c. Decide on exam date and location
4. **NCLEX/CGFNS preparation**
   a. Prep for exam
   b. Assess your Nursing and English skill
   c. Prepare and take TOEFL
   d. TOEFL Contact Information
   e. CGFNS demanding States
5. **License Verification**
   a. Verify license request
   b. Submit fingerprints
6. **Employment Verification**
   a. Submit employment verification
   b. Employment verification official form
7. **Employment and Sponsoring**
   a. Nursing vacancies & Sponsors 3-yr agreement
   b. Professional Recruiters & Hospitals
8. **USA Resumes and Video-Resumes**
   a. Prepare for webcam interviewing –
   b. Sell your skills and personality
9. **Working in USA – A new culture**
   a. Your family and You in USA
   b. Visas and Permanent Visa
   c. Purchasing a car and Your credit
   d. Your driver license – Safe driving in USA
   e. Social Security Not Just a Number
   f. Apt rentals and Utilities and more
10. **Buying Your First Home –USA Nurses Mortgages**
   a. Mortgages for Nurses Only – some States, like Florida offers favorable house buying loans for qualified nurses.

Becoming a Registered Nurse in United States

Step # 1 ~ Know All Steps and Sub-Steps

You're at step one to become a Registered Nurse or Professional Nurse in United States and that is to know all the steps needed, from A through Z, of the entire process. Take note of the main steps and the many sub-steps to successfully evaluate the process. Follow all steps minimizing any delays and additional expense.

Estimate Process Cost

Know the estimated cost of the entire process and of each step and plan accordingly. Plan for paying processes, such as credentialing of your education, preparing for exams, knowing when to pay and exactly how much covers the requested fee. Keep on top of your calendar. Missing a registration dateline for an exam may delay this for several months and/or lead you to lose your registration money. Even arriving late may to the examining center may cost you a delay and an additional fee.

Kwow Where You're going work or want to work – What State.

Knowing where – what State – in United States you want to work as a Registered Nurse must be decided before you take any Step # 2 Credentialing. Why? Several reasons. Each State has different requirements for foreign educated nurses seeking licensure as professional nurse or R.N. Some States allow licensure by 'Endorsement' while others only by "Examination". (The R.N. and Professional Nurse will be used interchangeably to denote a R.N. in this manual)

Step # 2~ Credentialing

Where do I begin? This is the most frequently question and confusing for most international nurses because there isn't one simple answer. The whole process from beginning to end may lead us to about "seven basic steps" and other countless sub-steps.

Refer to the Table of Content on this manual to stay on track and keep in mind all the steps.

Becoming a Registered Nurse in USA is a process with many steps and sub-steps. An understanding of the process and why each step is needed helps the internationally educated nurse visualize the all the needed steps from A – Z.

Let's begin with Step # 2 Credentialing or Educational Equivalencies. You will need to demonstrate to the State Board of Nursing where you anticipate to seek registration a nursing education similar or same followed American educated nurses. This step one has other sub-steps as follows below.

Credentials Evaluation Steps Information

Getting your accreditation through Credentialing Educational Services (CES) and/or any other authorized provider of these services usually takes time and it's expensive for most foreign educated nurses; considering, of course, the value of the American dollar of most foreign currencies, and the salaries earned by nurses outside USA. We suggest Joseph Silny in Miami, Florida for economical reasons. We not endorse any credentialing services and we're responsible for end results.

website: http://www.jsilny.com/html/foreign.htm

Most States will demand the submission of a CGFNS certification; some may demand that foreign educated nurses do credentialing through the State Board selected.

And all States required that nurses apply for the NCLEX exam and nurse registration.

Education Credentialing Services

Research on Internet for Educational Credentialing Services firms in USA that are officially designed National council State Boards of Nursing (www.NCSBN.org) to offer you their credentialing services. CGFNS is only one of many you can select from if wanting to save money and find the most affordable. Look for these firm in the Internet under "education credentials evaluation services".

Contact more than one firm; visit their website learning as much about the services. If in doubt ask as many questions as needed. If not sure simply do your credentialing through some of the traditional ones, however, expect to pay more for the same services and possibly wait longer.

Once you obtain the forms from the 'credentialing agency' or downloaded the form to initiate your credentialing you've done step one and sub-step one of credentialing and are ready to begin Step #2 or submitting a Educational Credentialing Request to a firm in USA.

Sub-Steps

Submitting your credentialing request begins with sub-step on for this process. That is, fill all the information requested on the 'credentialing request form'.

Some of the information is your own biographical information and while some of this information must is requested from you nursing school and the school will have to enter it on the form, including an official signature and a school stamp and/or official seal. This sub-step will be explained here soon.

- ❏ search for educational credentialing services and fill forms
- ❏ submit credentialing request and contact your nursing school
- ❏ mail the documentation yourself and follow up online with access ID #

Contacting Your Nursing School - Sub-Step of Step

You'll need to contact your nursing school and ask them fill the information requested by the credentialing educational services on their 'form you downloaded from their website' or the one you received via postal mail.

Be aware of the fact you cannot directly send your schooling transcription to any Education Credentialing Services (ECS).

SCHOOLS TRANSCRIPTS OR GRADES CANNOT BE SENT BY YOU TO CREDENTIALING INSTITUTIONS. ONLY YOUR NURSING SCHOOL CAN SEND YOUR GRADES.

Schools Transcripts or Grades Records

Your "school transcripts' must be sent out directly from your nursing school; however, your school in most cases will not know exactly what to send. Sending schools transcripts is not a practice for most schools outside United States. Some schools will know something about your need to present your equivalent nursing degree, but do not know the entire process in detail. It's up to you and for your own interest to look out for the completion of the process.

Therefore, you must: a) ill the information pertaining to your own biographical information, some information about the school you attended, the years you went to school, year of graduation and degree, etc., b) then take the form already filled, or mostly filled by you, and look for a school official in the Admissions and/or Registration department and explain your intentions of becoming a nurse in USA and c) you must seek the validating signature of the Registrar attesting that you're a graduate from that school.

High Schools Credentialing

Your education credentialing must include your high school education too. Al documents translated officially to English without exceptions.

All credentialing request forms have spaces for signature of school officials and official schools stamps. Both are part of filling a form completely.

Finally, have school official seal stamped on the enveloped used to send all the documents to the education credentialing services (ECS) institution. Make sure to bring an enveloped with pre-paid postage to the school you attended. Then have them close the envelope, seal it and then you place it in the mail box going out to USA.

Educational Credentialing Services Fees –

The fees you must pay for these services vary. Again CGFNS is only one of many institutions offering education credentialing services. Check other options is seeking to save money. On the web search for 'education credentialing service or foreign education credentialing services or credentialing services" and visit their websites for detailed information.

Make sure you send the fee requested by checking the firm's website. An incomplete fee will only delay the process or even nullify it if a correction is not submitted within the company's time frames. You may even lose all of the partial fee submitted. Most company's like CGFNS and many others may not refund your fees.

Submit the fee as requested by Money Order, Cashier Check or via credit card. We suggest credit cards that may stop a payment if something goes wrong. Other options are Paypal (visit www.paypal.com for a free account to buy or pay, or transfer).

Education Credentialing Services will confirm payment for their services acknowledging receipt of your request. Some of these firms may issue an Online Access Code allowing to follow up on the process of your credentialing. Ask the company selected if the option is offered. Online access allows to track the status of your credentialing. Credentialing services may take from thirty (30) to ninety (90) days. CGFNS takes ninety days or more.

Step # 2 RN Application Process

Once you have initiated your education credentialing process, you should initiate your Registered Nurse application process with the State in which you have decided to work. Why? Once the Education Credentialing Services company finishes your credentialing or equivalencies, the firm will send a certificate of a credentialing certificate to you and also one to the Nursing Board in the State where you are seeking to work. There must be an application submitted to a board of nursing"; to any board of nursing anywhere in USA by then.

In this case, the education credentialing services will send a 'credentialing certificate' to the nursing board you indicated in the Education Credentialing Services form prior to applying for a license. If no record of your application is on file with the nursing board, such credential certificate simply gets misplaced and/or archived somewhere.

Notice the processes are different and separate; each process done by two different institutions, both requiring separate processing fees. One is private company and the other a State institution. From the day that you send your request for education credentialing services to the time when your credentialing is done, you have from thirty to forty-five days to apply on time and have an application filed with a nursing home. So, about a month later after your credentialing request you must be getting ready to apply for a license as a Registered Nurse.

State Board Requirements

Prepare for the requirements of the nursing board. Visit the website of the nursing board of the State where you're seeking nurse registration. Visit www.NSCBN.org where you'll find a rosters and link to all nursing boards in USA.

Visit the web page of the nursing board of your selection and download their Registered Nurse Application forms. Some nursing boards will let you download the forms, others will expect a request and will mail out the forms to you.

Follow the nursing board requirements closely. Make sure you can comply with all the requirements. If you cannot comply with the expected requirements contact the nursing board emailing the Nursing Board Consultant or Supervisor listed on the web page. Follow through with phone call if you do not get a reply within seventy-two (72) hours.

Most nursing board have a Nurse Consultant that can help or listen or give instructions on issues about your application. Make sure to submit the correct 'application fee' and make it payable as indicated. Keep a copy of all documents and payments submitted for possible claim.

Sept # 3 License Request by Endorsement and/or Examination

Most internationally educated nurses, except USA territories like Puerto Rico, Guam ad Virgin Islands, will need to apply for license through CGFNS and/or NCLEX examinations. The Nursing Board in the State of your selection will look for your file for a 'education credentialing certificate', a verification of a license issued in your country, your English passing score – TOEFL or any other – before the Board can issue you an ATT or Authorization to Test, a written permission on your behalf to sit for the exam.

If you have satisfied at least the above three exigencies, the Nursing Board will issue you an ATT allowing to take the examination in most cases. Other pending issues, documents may be submitted, if missing. You should do every effort to submit all required documents at once.

The Board Nursing ATT

Once the Board of Nursing of your selected State issues an ATT on your behalf, you have now contact the Pearson-Vue the only authorized testing company allowed by the National Council of States of Nursing or NCSBN. You need to call Person Vue and register for the NCLEX exam. You must pay Person Vue the right to sit for the exam.

If you're seeking a Visa Screen through a CGFNS exam, you must contact CGFNS and schedule for a date, time and location of the exam. Allow yourself a least ninety (90) of exam preparation before attempting to take the test; unless you're absolutely sure that you do not need a 90-days preparation period.

Step # 4 Decide NCLEX or CFGNS or Both Exam

Preparing for the CGFNS or for the NCLEX is a common question. The CGFNS is a precursor test that predicts how well international nurse may do on the NCLEX if they take the CGFNS as preparation for the NCLEX. Internationally eduacated nurse may take the CGFNS if seeking a Visa Screen certificate.

Passing the CGFNS test for a Visa screen allows the nurse to obain, upon passing, a CGFNS Visa Screen certificate that allows the nurse to travel to USA with a temporary visa, then take the NCLEX in USA and apply for a Registered Nurse license. The CGFNS Visa Screen certificate allows nurses who pass the NCLEX to work on temporary upon getting a Registered License.

The CGFNS exam comprises a nursing exam similar to the NCLEX exam, and exams to assess the nurse English skills; both verbal and written skill. A standard score is expected for the verbal and written parts of the test. Nurse must pass both the written and verbal at the expected score to be issue a Visa Screen CGFNS certificate.

Visa Screen and CGFNS and FEES

The CGFNS exam must be requested from CGFNS, the only institution authorized to give out that exam. Upon passing the exam, a certificate is issued to the nurse who can in return seek a Temporary Visa from an American Consulate in her/his country of origin.

A Visa Screen allows internationally educated nurses taveling to USA and entering the country with such visa status. Upon passing NCLEX a status change is allowed by means of sponsorship by a hospital employer.

NCLEX Exam Only

Internationally educated nurse may opt for taking only the NCLEX exam in a country outside USA if offered or upon arrival to USA. Upon passing NCLEX in USA the nurse may apply for a temporary visa and the seek a visa adjustment – from temporary to permanent by means of sponsorship by a hospital employer.

NCLEX and CGFNS

Taking both the NCLEX and CGFNS means paying the exam fee for CGFNS and the exam fee for the NCLEX too.

CGFNS Demanded by Some States

Some States in USA demand that internationally educated nurse take the CGFNS and then also the NCLEX exam. Make you check the State's requirements to obtain a license as Registered Nurse. A list of States demanding the CGFNS exam is included in this guide.

Step # 5 The **VisaScreen** _Program_

The U.S. Citizenship and Immigration Services (USCIS) requires, under section 343 of the Illegal Immigration Reform and Immigrant Responsibility Act of 1996, that listed internationally educated health care professionals below, seeking temporary or permanent occupational visas as well as those who are seeking Trade NAFTA (TN) status, to first obtain a International Commission on Healthcare Professions _VisaScreen®_ certificate as part of the visa process. _VisaScreen®_ is administered by the International Commission on Healthcare Professions (ICHP) a division of CGFNS International.

- Registered Nurses
- Physical Therapists
- Occupational Therapists
- Physician Assistants
- Clinical Laboratory Technicians (Medical Technicians)
- Clinical Laboratory Scientists (Medical Laboratory Technologists)
- Speech Language Pathologists
- Audiologists
- Licensed Practical or Vocational Nurses

Fees for **VisaScreen**®_: Visa Credentials Assessment Fees_   **Dollars**

- _VisaScreen®_: Visa Credentials Assessment program initial certificate $498.00
  Valid for five years
- _VisaScreen®_: Reprocess an Expired Initial Order $128.00[1]
  Initial order was paid in full and applicant did not meet the
  requirements of the _VisaScreen®_ program within the first 12 months of
  placing the initial order and wants to continue with the service
- _VisaScreen®_: Expedited Review Services for applicants who have a $500.00
  Request for Evidence or deportation deadline
  See http://www.cgfns.org/sections/announcements/news/2009/06-22-
  09_expedited.shtml for futher information and contact instructions
  regarding this service.
- _VisaScreen®_: Visa Credentials Assessment program renewal certificate $250.00
  Valid for five years
- _VisaScreen®_: verification of certificate letter $75.00
  Verifies that a _VisaScreen®_ certificate was issued
- _VisaScreen®_: replacement certificate $100.00
  Replaces a missing original _VisaScreen®_ certificate (limit 1)

[1]Applicants will be given 12 months to meet the requirements of the program before the order is expired. Once an order that has been paid in full is expired, an applicant has up to one year (12 months) to apply to reprocess an expired order and pay the reprocess fee associated with this service. An applicant with an expired order that has not been paid in full must submit a new order with the full fee to continue the service. Reprocess orders will remain open for another 12 months starting from the date the reprocess order is placed. A reprocess order can only be placed for an expired order with full payment.

Step # 5 TOEFL Expected Scores

All applicants must have passing scores to meet program requirements for the specific CGFNS/ICHP service to which they have submitted an application.

Registered nurses, clinical laboratory scientists, speech language pathologists, audiologists and physicians assistants must submit a minimum total scores:

- ❑ 725 for TOEIC or 540 on the paper-based test, or

- ❑ 207 on the computer-based test for TOEFL, with 3.0 for TWE and 50 for TSE, or

- ❑ A minimum total score of 83 with 26 on the spoken for TOEFL iBT, or

- ❑ A minimum overall score of 6.5 with 7.0 on the spoken for the academic module of IELTS.

Institutions Names & Contact Information for TOEFL Examination

TOEFL, TWE, TSE and TOEFL iBT
TOEFL Services
Educational Testing Service (ETS)
PO Box 6151
Princeton, NJ 08541-6151 USA
Telephone: +1 (609) 771-7100 or +1 (877) 863-3546
Web site: http://www.ets.org

==TOEIC Testing

Program
Educational Testing Service (ETS)
Rosedale Road
Princeton, NJ 08540 USA
Telephone: +1 (800) 771-7170
Fax: +1 (609) 771-7111
Email: toeic@ets.org
Web site: http://www.ets.org/toeic

==IELTS

IELTS International
Suite 112
825 Colorado Boulevard
Los Angeles, CA 90041 USA
Telephone: +1 (323) 255-2771
Fax: +1 (323) 255-1261
Email: ielts@ieltsintl.org
Web site: http://www.ielts.org/

==

Step # 6 Your Nursing License Verification

Verification of your nursing license by the Nursing Institution claiming a registry for nursing professional takes time, money and patience. You must adhere to the requirements without exceptions.

Your license verification must be done through official institutions in your country and the State Board of Nursing you selected to get your license from in USA. The verification form is part of the application as registered nurse and is submitted to that institution holding your registration as professional nurse in your country. The form must be filled as indicated making sure all information requested if provided. The Ministry of Health, or Nursing Council, or State Board of Nursing holding the record of your registration as a Professional Nurse must sent such verification on your behalf to the Nursing Board you selected.

License Verification Sub-Steps

Take the 'license verification page' that you downloaded or was sent to you to anyone of the institution named above. In most cases in non-English speaking countries the information will not be entered correctly, or the information may not be complete.

We suggest you create a draft of the same form, fill it correctly in pencil and take your filled and a blank form have the personnel at the institution follow your draft as a sample. This small effort form you will avoid sending out an 'incorrectly' filled form or one missing the information requested. This sub-step alone may delay the process and increase your cost.

Take a pre-paid and pre-addressed enveloped where once the 'license verification' form is completed your institution simply put it in the mail on your behalf. We suggest you request a copy of what was sent out in case the document never arrives. If you paid for this service keeping a copy may save paying for the whole process again.

Step # 7 Your FingerPrints Submission

The application package sent out to you may bring the 'fingerprints card'. This a police 'fingerprints' card with the "stamped" name of the Board of Nursing sending you the application package. The 'fingerprints card' must be filled correctly to have any validity or to useful to the authorities running the fingerprints comparison – usually the FBI in Washington. If the prints are unreadable for any reason, a second an better print is requested after several after the arrival of the your 'fingerprints' to the FBI quarters.

Take the 'fingerprints' to the police station or institution where fingerprinting is done. Explain to the 'technicians' the need to rolled the finger thoroughly to imprint the best fingerprints on the card to avoid a second print. Most technicians know how to correctly do this, but is good practice to let them know and avoid this delay. In some countries 'fingerprints' are done by 'private investigators' using unofficial or poor quality ink that smudges over the card with unclear prints.

Step # 8 Employment Verification Submission Form

The application package sent out to you will have an 'employment verification' form that must be filled by a Human Resources Department using that form only. Most internationally educated nurse do not submit an 'employment verification' form. Employment Verification form are submitted by nurses seeking licensure by endorsement and not by examination. The employment verification requirement do not apply to you if your seeking licensure by examination.

Step # 9 Working in USA ~ Employment and Nursing Vacancies

Employing yourself as Registered or Professional Nurse in USA will be rewarding for you and your family in many ways. Working as a nurse and being a nurse in USA is different in many ways than what foreign educated nurses know.

Most of the questions you may have now are answered in the following sections below. For the foreign educated nurse (Registered Nurse in USA) transitioning to a new country, like USA, and learning about a new culture and adapting to new employment and environment may represent great challenges. On the other hand, those challanges are not unrewarded.

The foreign educated nurse will find that all nurses in USA are held in great esteem in their communities, and deserve great respect and are well compensated for their education and experience.

Nursing has evolved as a profession of many specialized areas with a broader spectrum of opportunities to foreign and native nurses without distinction of gender, race, political association, or religious belief and/or age.

However, all nurses in USA face great responsibilities as well; their work is closely monitored and is expected of them only the best intervention, every minute, always; there is no room for error, or negligence when taking care and intervening patients.

As new arrival from another nation, a nurse encounters obstacles seemingly insurmountable at first, but as time goes by, foreign nurses adapt to new employment, to new healthcare intervention protocols, and soon before it's realized they too become part of the American Dream like millions more from all over the world.

Our life style and standard of living is advance and most of our citizen are from middle class, or working class, the most numerous of the social classes. There is no accentuated distinction of social classes. We're simply most of us as working class, and we're very proud of that heritage.

Once you have your USA Nursing Licensure, you may apply to become a Permanent Resident, and 5 years after residing in the country, you have the option of adopting the American citizenship.

Green Card Holders

As a Green Card holder you and your family can live in the United States forever and lead a secure and comfortable life lifestyle. Your children can enjoy free schooling till the age of 18. You would also get to feel at home with all major American cities having immigrants from most countries of the world.

Step # 10 Nursing Vacancies Salaries and Benefits in USA Hospitals

The USA Labor Department oversees your employees' rights and employment conditions making sure you are paid "prevailing wages".

Most employers offer a benefits package for you and family as the case may be. Your base hourly wage will be determined after your hospital placement and will be based on the local prevailing wage of nurses in your location.

Base hourly wages generally range from $18 to $30 but are always well above the average salary for any worker in the United States. Higher salaries are possible for specialties and based on years of experience. Employers also provides you with free health insurance and other benefits including paid vacation, professional liability insurance and workers compensation insurance.

The graph below depicts nursing wages in relation to other professions in USA

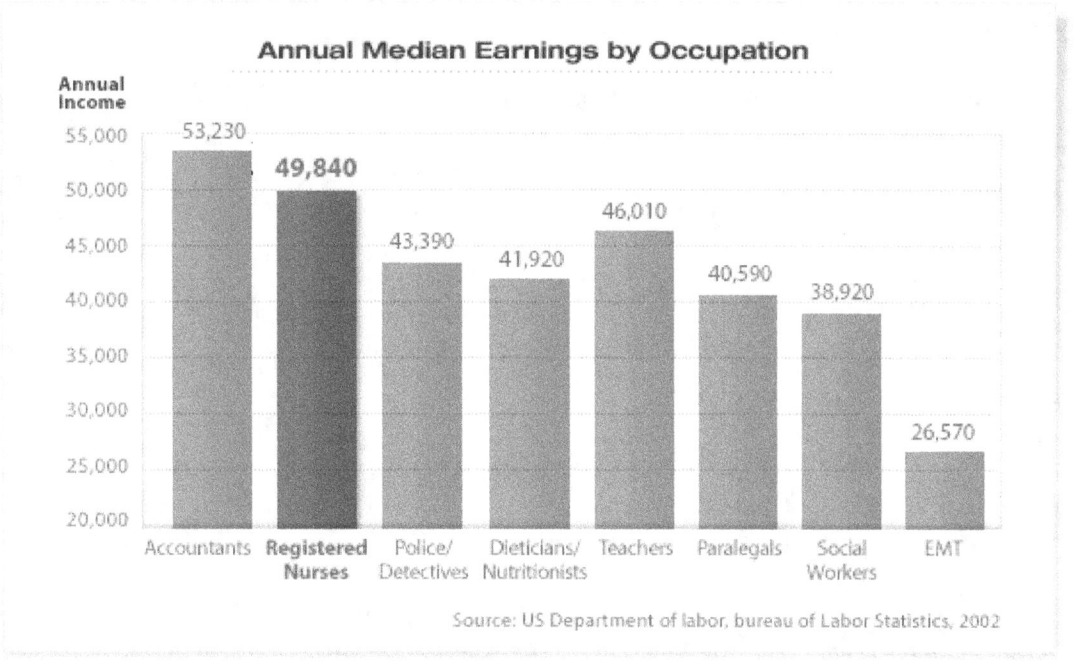

All wages paid by employers are those who prevail in local and national markets and employer will pay you salaries closely similar to those of other RN's every considered the same for skills set, experience and education, as set forth by the Dept of Labor. Wages will be commensurate with your experience and specialty in most cases.

13

Shift and Number of Working Hours

You will be working a minimum of three 12 hour shifts a week amounting to 36 hours/week. You will be paid an overtime wage of 1.5 times your base salary for any hours over 40 worked in one week.

You may also be paid a night differential or added wages per hours depending on the location of your placement and shift. Night shift and rotating shifts are common for most new arrivals. Every other weekend off is also the norm in most hospitals.

Other benefits include medical, dental and visual insurance for you and your family; contribution to insurance plans is the norm in most hospitals; however, healthcare facilities pay most of the premium.

Professional Healthcare Recruiting Firms

By searching in the Internet under 'healthcare recruiters' you will identify those recruiting firms and/or employer who offer the best benefits and/or stipends when they recruit you and represent you in all processes of your relocation and employment in USA.

Many offer sponsoring opportunities through hospital employers, while the recruiting may offer you airfare, relocation support, free rental and/or housing. Also vehicle purchasing assistance and work hard and honestly on your behalf; however, all these affiliations are optional and not guaranteed in anyway.

We suggest you contact them via the Internet and check their recruiting history by asking for references from other nurses and from hospitals working with them.

Visa Processing on Your Behalf

Once you have a license as Registered Nurse and are holding an 'occupational visa' under the nursing class, you may file your I-140 petition (immigrant visa petition). You may file the petition by yourself or through immigration lawyer, or a hospital lawyer if offered that opportunity.

Non-Profit organizations representing foreign nationals from many countries may be an option. Sometimes the visa process is handled by a sponsoring hospital through third party lawyer or their own lawyers.

Expect to sign a minimum of two years agreement in lieu of sponsorship by an employer. This means two things; one, you have assured employment for at least two years and two you must work for that employer for two years. This is usually a good deal for most nurses. The two years of employment will provide the initial training to secure employment anywhere after that at prevailing wages commensurate with your experience.

Seeking Employment with a Hospital in USA

Submit a CurriculumVitae or Resume with a professional presentation and Word format to employers. Use a current USA Resume formats looking into samples on the Internet. We suggest visiting www.imedcorp.net where interviewing sessions and resume formats are posted with a 'interviewing session' as a good example of positive interviewing.

Consider submitting a home made Video-Resume using a webcam to sell your skills and personality and enhance your probabilities of being hired and offered sponsorship. Keep in mind that other foreign educated nurses, like yourself, may be competing for the same vacancy. Make the best impression, the first time.

Do a professional presentation of yourself using a well rehearsed format. Use good lighting and clean, well kept surrounding and background when doing this. A good picture – video – is worth a thousand words. Be sincere about your skills and abilities, but make good emphasis on your best skills. Demonstrate a great motivation to relocate 'permanently' seeking to become an American citizens too.

Many hospitals may consider your sponsorship of foreign educated already licensed in USA. Others simply refuse for many corporate reasons and lengthy processes. Most employers require nurses to have at least 2 years of experience before sponsoring a nurse; nevertheless, many other employers will considered bright recent grads who have passed the CGFNS and NCLEX exams.

You and Your Family

Cultural transitioning and cultural shock go hand on hand. You and your family member will enter a new culture with many things to learn and adapt to within a short time frame; this specially true of yourself.

Your work setting and responsibilities will demand your rapid transition. You're now a Registered Nurse on the floor and many will be the expectations of your healthcare team.

At the same time your family members, husband, children or parents will transitioning too. Learn as much as you can about the USA culture, social mores, foods, etc. Watching American television offers a rapid cultural understanding of the American ways of life without actually making an immersion; that comes later as time goes by.

Purchasing Your First Car and Your Credit

Most Americans drive to work everyday despite most movies show thousand of people commuting in NY or CA. You most likely will need to buy a car and with that need to buy a car, you will also need either some cash to buy a second hand car or credit to buy a brand new car from the dealer. Most credits histories from foreign countries aren't acceptable by local car dealers and other merchants. Plan saving for used car. Check your Internet for "Used Car Dealers, Florida, Miami, USA" as an example to see used cars and prices.

Your Driver License and Safe Driving in USA

Many foreign are do not driving in USA as challenging as driving in Mexico city or Mumbay, India. Others do find driving here challenging because our may highways and signs and police enforcement of traffic laws.

Your driver license as foreign national may be good for driving for about three months. Check with the State Division of Drivers License to make sure you're within the law as you drive, or contact them to get one. The Drivers License division offers the booklets you may need to prepare for your written and on-the-road practice exam.

Before you can drive your own vehicle and proudly show to work with a brand new car, you need an insurance policy too. Most dealers arrange for that before you drive away with their car, but the monthly insurance bill is your responsibility. Ask all the questions about anything you don't know. Don't shy about asking questions.

The Social Security – More than just a number

Your "Social Security' number is simply a number associated to your name and which your employment – income you earned and taxed – income is placed in scrow for your future use. If unemployment or disability comes to you for any reason, you may received financial assistance from the State of residency – where you're employed and live – for some time until you recover or are employed again. Most people are taxed at the rate ofa about 15% per paycheck for your own welfare in the near future.

Upon your arrival to your State, visit your nearest 'Social Security' office to request your own number and card. This card is one of our official identifications, along with driver license since we do not carry a national identity card – it does not exist yet.Your Alien Registration is your most common identification for foreign nationals.

Apartment Rental and Utilities

When renting an apartment you will be required to produce an identification and for sure a 'Social Security Card' amongst other requirements. In some places even your credit history if you're a local. Rentals are usually contacted for at least 12 months and breaking the contract may result in paying the rent even though you left.

Once you have rented your own apartment and ready to move, you need to contact the electricity power supplying company and open an account. A deposit is required for some time and then refunded with interest.

Buying Your Home with Mortgages for Nurse Only

When you ready to purchase your first home – possibly within two years from arrival to USA – explore the mortgages offered to nurses only. There is a program offering nurses zero interest and no credit history to buy any home, anywhere, for any price range as long as you can pay for the obligation. For nurses only. Welcome to USA..!

USA Hospitals Seeking Nurses

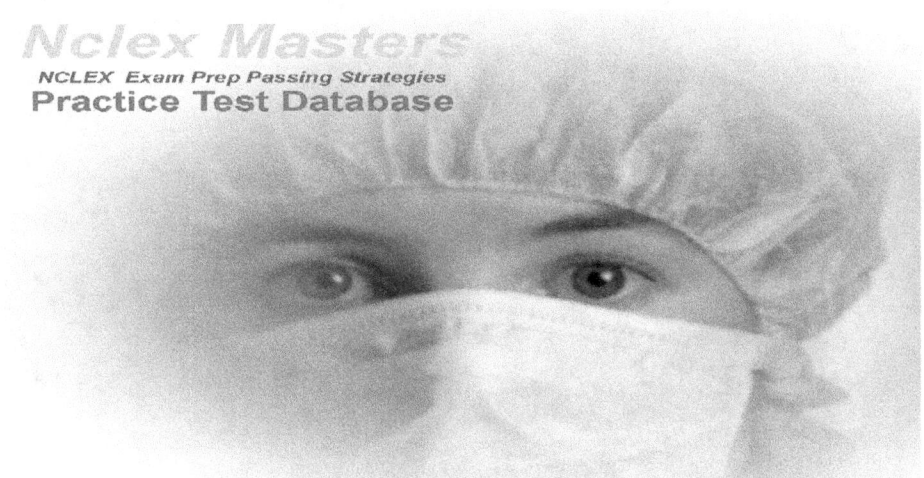

Nclex Masters
NCLEX Exam Prep Passing Strategies
Practice Test Database

www.Nclex-masters.net

Free Online exam practice

Hospital Name	Beds	City	State	ZIP
60th Medical Group - David Grant USAF Medical Center	0	Travis Air Force Base	CA	94535
Agnews Developmental Center	24	San Jose	CA	95134-2299
Alameda Hospital	95	Alameda	CA	94501
Alhambra Hospital Medical Center	144	Alhambra	CA	91801
Alta Bates Summit Medical Center - Alta Bates Campus	549	Berkeley	CA	94705
Alta Bates Summit Medical Center - Herrick Campus	0	Berkeley	CA	94704
Alta Bates Summit Medical Center - Summit Campus	402	Oakland	CA	94609
Alvarado Hospital Medical Center	306	San Diego	CA	92120

Hospital Name	Beds	City	State	ZIP
Alvarado Parkway Institute	66	La Mesa	CA	91942
Anaheim General Hospital	143	Anaheim	CA	92804
Anaheim Memorial Medical Center	223	Anaheim	CA	92801
Antelope Valley Hospital	420	Lancaster	CA	93534
Arden Wood	13	San Francisco	CA	94116
Arrowhead Regional Medical Center	373	Colton	CA	92324
Arroyo Grande Community Hospital	65	Arroyo Grande	CA	93420
Atascadero State Hospital	0	Atascadero	CA	93422
Aurora Charter Oak Hospital	95	Covina	CA	91724
Aurora Las Encinas Hospital	122	Pasadena	CA	91107
Aurora San Diego Hospital	80	San Diego	CA	92128
Aurora Vista Del Mar Hospital	79	Ventura	CA	93001
Bakersfield Heart Hospital	47	Bakersfield	CA	93308
Bakersfield Memorial Hospital	307	Bakersfield	CA	93301
Banner Lassen Medical Center	25	Susanville	CA	96130
Barlow Respiratory Hospital	105	Los Angeles	CA	90026
Barlow Respiratory Hospital at Presbyterian Intercommunity Hospital	0	Whittier	CA	90602
Barlow Respiratory Hospital at Valley Presbyterian Hospital	0	Van Nuys	CA	91405
Barstow Community Hospital	50	Barstow	CA	92311
Barton Memorial Hospital	119	South Lake Tahoe	CA	96150
Hospital Name	Beds	City	State	ZIP
6th Medical Group - MacDill Air Force Base	0	MacDill Air Force Base	FL	33621
96th Medical Group - United States Air Force Regional Hospital	0	Eglin Air Force Base	FL	32542
A.G. Holley State Hospital	100	Lantana	FL	33462
All Children's Hospital	216	Saint Petersburg	FL	33701
Apalachee Center, Inc.	24	Tallahassee	FL	32308
Arnold Palmer Hospital for Children	0	Orlando	FL	32806
Atlantic Shores Hospital	72	Fort Lauderdale	FL	33308
Aventura Hospital and Medical Center	407	Aventura	FL	33180

Hospital Name	Beds	City	State	ZIP
Baptist Hospital	492	Pensacola	FL	32501
Baptist Hospital of Miami	584	Miami	FL	33176
Baptist Medical Center Beaches	146	Jacksonville Beach	FL	32250
Baptist Medical Center Downtown	699	Jacksonville	FL	32207
Baptist Medical Center Nassau	54	Fernandina Beach	FL	32034
Baptist Medical Center South	0	Jacksonville	FL	32258
Bartow Regional Medical Center	72	Bartow	FL	33830
Bascom Palmer Eye Institute	56	Miami	FL	33136
Bay Medical	413	Panama City	FL	32401
Bay Pines VA Healthcare System	0	Bay Pines	FL	33744
Bayfront Medical Center	382	Saint Petersburg	FL	33701
Bert Fish Medical Center	112	New Smyrna Beach	FL	32169
Bethesda Memorial Hospital	401	Boynton Beach	FL	33435
Blake Medical Center	383	Bradenton	FL	34209
Boca Raton Community Hospital	400	Boca Raton	FL	33486
Brandon Regional Hospital	367	Brandon	FL	33511
Brooks Rehabilitation Hospital	143	Jacksonville	FL	32216
Brooksville Regional Hospital	244	Brooksville	FL	34601
Broward General Medical Center	640	Fort Lauderdale	FL	33316
Calhoun-Liberty Hospital	15	Blountstown	FL	32424
Campbellton-Graceville Hospital	25	Graceville	FL	32440
Cape Canaveral Hospital	150	Cocoa Beach	FL	32931
Cape Coral Hospital	305	Cape Coral	FL	33990
Capital Regional Medical Center	198	Tallahassee	FL	32308

Hospital Name	Beds	City	State	ZIP
375th Medical Group - Scott Air Force Base Medical Center	0	Scott Air Force Base	IL	62225
Abraham Lincoln Memorial Hospital	25	Lincoln	IL	62656
Adventist Bolingbrook Medical Center	0	Bolingbrook	IL	60440
Adventist GlenOaks Hospital	159	Glendale Heights	IL	60139

Hospital Name	Beds	City	State	ZIP
Adventist Hinsdale Hospital	327	Hinsdale	IL	60521
Adventist La Grange Memorial Hospital	177	La Grange	IL	60525
Advocate Bethany Hospital	84	Chicago	IL	60624
Advocate Christ Medical Center	642	Oak Lawn	IL	60453
Advocate Condell Medical Center	253	Libertyville	IL	60048
Advocate Good Samaritan Hospital	326	Downers Grove	IL	60515
Advocate Good Shepherd Hospital	181	Barrington	IL	60010
Advocate Illinois Masonic Medical Center	354	Chicago	IL	60657
Advocate Lutheran General Hospital	584	Park Ridge	IL	60068
Advocate South Suburban Hospital	289	Hazel Crest	IL	60429
Advocate Trinity Hospital	179	Chicago	IL	60617
Alexian Brothers Behavioral Health Hospital	137	Hoffman Estates	IL	60169
Alexian Brothers Medical Center	387	Elk Grove Village	IL	60007
Alexian Rehabilitation Hospital	0	Elk Grove Village	IL	60007
Alton Memorial Hospital	152	Alton	IL	62002
Alton Mental Health Center	24	Alton	IL	62002
Anderson Hospital	130	Maryville	IL	62062
Aurora Chicago Lakeshore Hospital	113	Chicago	IL	60640
Blessing Hospital	287	Quincy	IL	62305
BroMenn Regional Medical Center	200	Normal	IL	61761
Cancer Treatment Centers of America at Midwestern Regional Medical Center	69	Zion	IL	60099
Carle Foundation Hospital	259	Urbana	IL	61801
Carlinville Area Hospital	25	Carlinville	IL	62626
Centegra Hospital - McHenry	183	McHenry	IL	60050
Centegra Hospital - Woodstock	145	Woodstock	IL	60098
Centegra Specialty Hospital - Woodstock	0	Woodstock	IL	60098
Central DuPage Hospital	313	Winfield	IL	60190
CGH Medical Center	92	Sterling	IL	61081
Chicago Read Mental Health Center	24	Chicago	IL	60634

l Name	Beds	City	State	ZIP
Abilene Regional Medical Center	205	Abilene	TX	79606
Acadia Abilene	32	Abilene	TX	79602
Allegiance Behavioral Health Center Of Plainview	25	Plainview	TX	79072
Allegiance Specialty Hospital of Kilgore	66	Kilgore	TX	75662
Amarillo VA Health Care System - Thomas E. Creek VA Medical Center	0	Amarillo	TX	79106
Angleton Danbury Medical Center	62	Angleton	TX	77515
Anson General Hospital	27	Anson	TX	79501
Apex Hospital - Houston	18	Houston	TX	77004
Apex Hospital - Katy	0	Katy	TX	77494
Arlington Rehabilitation Hospital	24	Arlington	TX	76012
Atlanta Memorial Hospital	65	Atlanta	TX	75551
Atrium Medical Center at Corinth	10	Corinth	TX	76208
Austin Lakes Hospital at Saint David's Pavilion	48	Austin	TX	78705
Austin State Hospital	299	Austin	TX	78751
Austin Surgical Hospital	23	Austin	TX	78746
Ballinger Memorial Hospital	16	Ballinger	TX	76821
Baptist Medical Center	1,439	San Antonio	TX	78205
Baptist Saint Anthony's Hospital	442	Amarillo	TX	79106
Baylor All Saints Medical Center at Fort Worth	508	Fort Worth	TX	76104
Baylor Institute for Rehabilitation	86	Dallas	TX	75246
Baylor Jack and Jane Hamilton Heart and Vascular Hospital	49	Dallas	TX	75226
Baylor Medical Center at Frisco	68	Frisco	TX	75034
Baylor Medical Center at Garland	214	Garland	TX	75042
Baylor Medical Center at Irving	193	Irving	TX	75061
Baylor Medical Center at Southwest Fort Worth	0	Fort Worth	TX	76132
Baylor Medical Center at Trophy Club	20	Trophy Club	TX	76262
Baylor Medical Center at Waxahachie	57	Waxahachie	TX	75165
Baylor Regional Medical Center at Grapevine	220	Grapevine	TX	76051
Baylor Regional Medical Center at Plano	101	Plano	TX	75093
Baylor Specialty Hospital - Dallas	61	Dallas	TX	75204

I Name	Beds	City	State	ZIP
Baylor University Medical Center at Dallas	853	Dallas	TX	75246

For employment with any of the above USA hospitals

Hospital Name	Beds	City	State	ZIP
A.L. Lee Memorial Hospital	67	Fulton	NY	13069
A.O. Fox Hospital	259	Oneonta	NY	13820
Adirondack Medical Center	157	Saranac Lake	NY	12983
Albany Medical Center	600	Albany	NY	12208
Albany Medical Center - South Clinical Campus	20	Albany	NY	12208
Albany Memorial Hospital	165	Albany	NY	12204
Albany VA Medical Center	0	Albany	NY	12208
Alice Hyde Medical Center	151	Malone	NY	12953
Amsterdam Memorial Healthcare	199	Amsterdam	NY	12010
Arms Acres	0	Carmel	NY	10512
Arnot Ogden Medical Center	238	Elmira	NY	14905
Auburn Memorial Hospital	271	Auburn	NY	13021
Bath VA Medical Center	0	Bath	NY	14810
Bellevue Hospital Center	912	New York	NY	10016
Bellevue Woman's Care Center	40	Niskayuna	NY	12309
Benedictine Hospital	169	Kingston	NY	12401
Bertrand Chaffee Hospital	104	Springville	NY	14141
Beth Israel Medical Center - Kings Highway Division	0	Brooklyn	NY	11239
Beth Israel Medical Center - Petrie Division	975	New York	NY	10003
Binghamton General Hospital	509	Binghamton	NY	13903
Blythedale Children's Hospital	0	Valhalla	NY	10595
Bon Secours Community Hospital	183	Port Jervis	NY	12771
Bronx Children's Psychiatric Center	0	Bronx	NY	10461
Bronx Psychiatric Center	362	Bronx	NY	10461
Bronx-Lebanon Hospital Center - Concourse Division	0	Bronx	NY	10457

Hospital Name	Beds	City	State	ZIP
Bronx-Lebanon Hospital Center - Fulton Division	579	Bronx	NY	10456-3402
Brookhaven Memorial Hospital Medical Center	258	East Patchogue	NY	11772
Brooklyn Children's Center	0	Brooklyn	NY	11233
Brooks Memorial Hospital	64	Dunkirk	NY	14048
Brylin Hospitals	88	Buffalo	NY	14209
Buffalo General Hospital	1,241	Buffalo	NY	14203
Buffalo Psychiatric Center	254	Buffalo	NY	14213
Calvary Hospital	225	Bronx	NY	10461
Canandaigua VA Medical Center	0	Canandaigua	NY	14424

For employment with any of the above USA hospitals